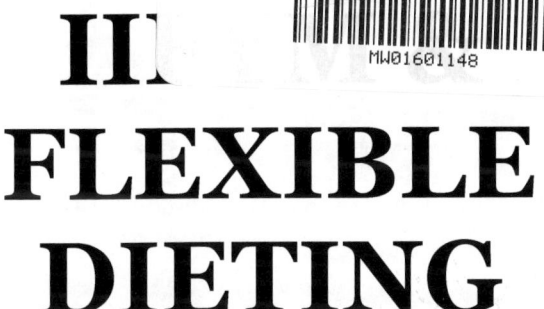

# II
# FLEXIBLE
# DIETING

**Beginners Step-By-Step "If It Fits Your Macros"**

**Diet Guide - Quickly & Easily Lose Weight And**

**Burn Fat By Counting Your Macros.**

By *Jennifer Louissa*

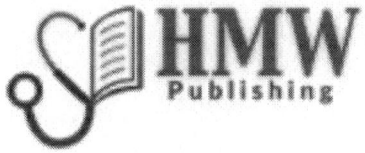

For more great books visit:

**HMWPublishing.com**

# Download another book for Free

I want to thank you for purchasing this book and offer you another book (just as long and valuable as this book), "Health & Fitness Mistakes You Don't Know You're Making", completely free.

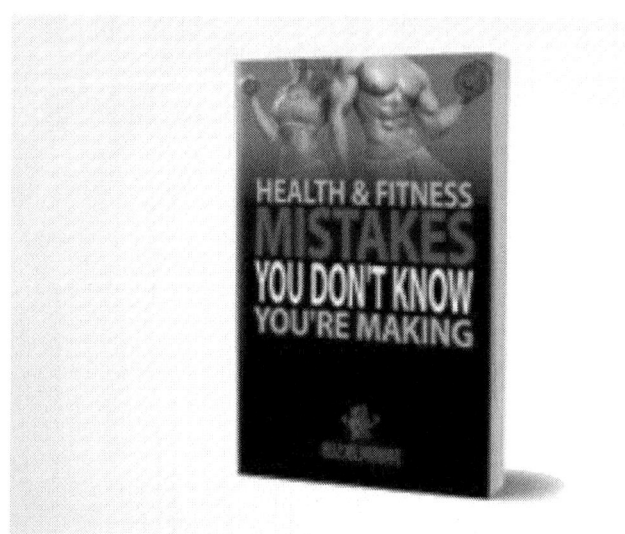

Visit the link below to signup and receive it:

**www.hmwpublishing.com/gift**

In this book, I will break down the most common health & fitness mistakes, you are probably committing right now, and I will reveal how you can easily get in the best shape of your life!

In addition to this valuable gift, you will also have an opportunity to get our new books for free, enter giveaways, and receive other valuable emails from me. Again, visit the link to sign up:

**www.hmwpublishing.com/gift**

# TABLE OF CONTENTS

# Introduction

I want to thank you and congratulate you for purchasing the "IFYM Flexible Dieting & Counting Macros" book. The best fat loss *strategy*, in my experience, has been IIFYM (If It Fits Your Macros). Another name for this revolutionary way of eating is *Flexible Dieting* or simply *Counting Your Macros*. IIFYM has been used for years now. Both people who aim to lose fat or build muscle use it.

IIFYM & Flexible Dieting offers anyone the opportunity to tailor their diets to their favourite nutritious foods, mixing their favourite treats every day, and still make progress towards their fitness goals.

Is it realistic to say that you're never going to eat ice cream, burgers or pizza again? Are your only carbs going to come from veggies (I can't even stand the thought)? Are you going to trade all these so-called "dirty foods" out for meals consisting of chicken, brown rice, broccoli and maybe some sweet potatoes if you're lucky? My guess is probably not. That approach to weight loss can cause you to have a total binge day in the future. Not only would your diet be strict and boring, but you'll most likely gain back all the "strict diet" weight you lost in the first place.

IIFYM is also a method of dieting used to improve body composition by tracking macronutrients (macros). Three main macros are traditionally accounted for: protein, carbs, and fats. By monitoring macros, you naturally track your calories as well.

This way of dieting has been gaining vast popularity and chances are you've heard of it. If you've done any research on IIFYM & Flexible Dieting in the past you've, perhaps, realized that no foods are off limits. No food groups are labeled good or bad for you. What matters, in this style of dieting, is if your macro budget has room for the foods you want to eat. If so then you're in the clear, but more on that soon.

So how did this type of dieting come about? Well, bodybuilder's in the old days simply got tired of eating the same bland foods when preparing for a competition. They ate the kind of food that scares people away from attempting to lose weight in the first place! These boring, clean meals, included chicken, broccoli, rice, veggies, eggs, and well—you get the picture. There's no denying that this *"bro science"* approach to dieting works, but the real question is: is it worth it? After years of making bodybuilders miserable If It Fits Your Macros was born. IIFYM is thus a way to improve one's body composition by not solely relying on clean foods. Thanks again for purchasing this book, I hope you enjoy it and please don't forget to leave us an honest review!

Also, before you get started, I recommend you **joining our email newsletter** to receive updates on any upcoming new book releases or promotions. You can sign-up for free, and as a bonus, you will receive a free gift. Our *"Health & Fitness Mistakes You Don't Know You're Making"* book! This book has been written to demystify, expose the top do's and don'ts and to finally equip you with the information you need to get in the best shape of your life. Due to the overwhelming amount of mis-information and lies told by magazines and self-proclaimed "gurus", it's becoming harder and harder to get reliable information to get in shape. As opposed to having to go through dozens of biased, unreliable and untrustworthy sources to get your health & fitness information. Everything you need to help you has been broken down in this book for you to easily follow and to immediately get results to achieve your desired fitness goals in the shortest amount of time.

Once again, to join our free email newsletter and to receive a free copy of this valuable book, please visit the link and signup now: **www.hmwpublishing.com/gift**

# CHAPTER 1: WHAT IS "IIFYM"?

A common misconception of IIFYM (If It Fits Your Macros) is that it's just an excuse to eat junk food every day. This is not the case. Contrary to popular belief, IIFYM is not about eating pop tarts for breakfast every day. Unlike traditional diets, you have the *option* to eat what you want, when you want, if you make it fit into your eating plans.

Although the option to eat so-called greasy foods (pizza, burgers, ice cream, cookies, etc.) exists, you certainly don't have to part take in it. The edge that IIFYM dieting has over traditional dieting is its flexibility. This flexibility offers you the ability to improve your body composition without having to be perfect or strict with your diet behaviour.

There's no reason to be super strict or go on a fad diet. The fad diet approach never last and there seems to be one coming out every other month! Specifically, there's no need for dramatic, and unhealthy, calorie restrictions or any elimination of any particular macronutrient (this includes low-carb approaches). Once you understand the fundamentals of calories and macros, you'll have a better understanding of why hardcore and fad diets fall short.

Although IIFYM can be used for gaining lean muscle mass, *IIFYM: The Ultimate Beginner's Guide* is tailored towards implementing IIFYM for fat loss. This style of eating is more realistic for people who want to lose fat and enjoy the process.

## The benefits of IIFYM:

- Realistic & psychologically beneficial;
- A long-term approach a healthy lifestyle:
- Compatible with the energy balance law (more on this in Chapter 2).
- Flexible food choices;
- It works perfectly with My Fitness Pal (IIFYM-friendly smartphone app).

This approach to fat loss is centered around knowing your macros and hitting your daily macro goals.

My Fitness Pal is the number one tool that makes IIFYM easy to implement.

The following chapters are the fundamentals that you'll need to know to integrate IIFYM into your daily routine.

# CHAPTER 2: DEBUNKING THE MYTHS

As with anything new and different, there are going to be pros and cons as well as many misconceptions – and a few distorted myths. In this chapter, we're going to sort those out so the truth will shine through.

## Debunking Myth #1:

## You can gorge on junk food and lose weight.

The flexible dieting plan is an inclusive plan. You will not be told to abstain from any specific food groups. Because of this surprising (and different) concept, the myth is that a person can eat all the junk food they want, which of course is entirely erroneous.

Let's go back and refer to your personal goals. Do you want to achieve:

- Weight loss?

- Weight maintenance?

- Muscle toning?

- Muscle building?

Common sense says if you want to build muscles, it's not going to happen on a steady diet of ice cream and chocolate chip cookies. Plus the fact that fiber is missing.

This myth may have emerged due to online blogs, articles, and ads that have to do with flexible dieting. What's the most common graphics featured on those sites? Donuts, candy, pizza, and maybe a Big Mac.

The reason for this is because it indeed is good news that a diet no longer has to be torture and agony. After all, if you can improve your body composition while still enjoying some junk food, let's tell the world – even if it has to involve lots of junk food pictures.

But let's return to reality. Flexible dieters eat a diet composed of whole food sources with a dash of fun indulgences on the side. The wise, flexible dieter still makes it a goal to hit their daily macronutrient intakes because health is always important.

## Debunking Myth #2:

## Clean foods are the only healthy foods so flexible dieting cannot be healthy.

Granted a great deal of the American diet is made up of processed foods, some of which are not indeed food at all but simply manufactured products that have little nutritional value. However, to get caught up in the fallacy that *clean foods* are the only *healthy foods* merely is another trap.

To follow that line of thinking we have to return to the excellent food vs. bad food mentality. What good can ever come out of making certain foods *off-limits?* Because the moment you give in to temptation and eat foods that are on the no-no list, the guilt issues resurface. And who needs those?

Various studies have shown that just as soon as a particular food is restricted, the desire for it grows. Even if that person never really had a craving for that food before the restriction. Difficult to explain, but it's true. We are psychological beings, and this is how the human mind (and emotions) operates.

## Debunking Myth #3:

## Flexible diets lack structure (they're all over the place).

This myth is quite easily explained. It merely arises because habitual dieters are so accustomed to the shackles of a restricted diet. They have confused limitations with structure. They're not the same.

Indeed, flexible dieting is a structured method, but without the restraints and restrictions. The successful flexible dieter will take the time to consider what food source – and in what amount – is the best for the activities of this day. Tomorrow may be different.

## Debunking Myth #4:

## Flexible dieters are looking for an easy way out – they're lazy.

This fourth and final myth, to me, is the most humorous. To follow the logic of this thinking, one has to assume that jumping from one restrictive fad diet to another while trying to remember which foods are restricted on which diet, while excitedly awaiting the Saturday night cheat meal, is considered a productive way to spend your time. I don't think so.

It does require a good deal of planning for the flexible dieter to find the foods that fit with their daily macronutrients. The difference here is that you are thinking for yourself, rather than having some diet guru tell you how to make it work for you. You may want to learn more about nutrition, food, and macronutrients. Your incentive will be stronger, simply because you're not entering the dieter's torture chamber. You're discovering what's best for you and your goals.

In the next chapter we're going to do just that – take a closer look at macronutrients.

# CHAPTER 3: FLEXIBLE DIETING VS. STRICT DIETING

In this chapter, we want to take a close look at how the typical strict diets/fad diets compare to the flexible dieting method. We want to look at three separate areas:

- 1) Body.

- 2) Mind (emotions).

- 3) Lifestyle.

## *1) Comparison of Your Body:*

## Strict / Fad Diets

Dieters who have spent years on the fad-dieting roller coaster often cease to appreciate the complexity of their body and how it functions. Misplaced priorities put many aspects of health and wellness on the back burner. This means that the body can be abused and health can be compromised in the quest for that *perfect* body weight. (As mentioned earlier, *perfection* is impossible to attain.)

The stopping and starting of various types of diets put stress on the digestive system, as well as vital organs such as the heart and liver.

Likewise, switching restrictive diets can also be harmful. This happens when a discouraged dieter moves from one diet to another in search of the secret to weight loss. Diets that forbid one or more food groups can cause nutritional deficiencies and throw the body entirely out of whack.

Another dangerous effect on chronic dieters is the increased inability to recognize the body's signals of hunger and fullness. Those who suffer from this *dieting side effect* report that they can go for long periods of time without any sense of being hungry. But then, once they start eating again, their appetite goes entirely out of control.

By its very essence, the fad diet is an on-again, off-again pattern, which as mentioned, creates some hardships on overall health.

# Flexible Diet

The flexible diet can hardly even be called a diet. In direct contrast to fad diets, this points to a *lifestyle* rather than a quick fix. This means less stress on the body and the body's systems.

Remember we stressed that the flexible diet starts with *your* goals and purposes, not just some one-size-fits-all type of diet.

So what is your goals? Is it:

. Weight loss?

. Weight maintenance?

. Muscle toning?

. Muscle building?

Whichever it is, this is where you begin. From there you move into which foods best work to achieve these goals. If you get most of your daily calories (let's say 80%) from mostly unprocessed, nutrient-dense foods, then with the flexible diet you can feel free to fill the remaining 20% with the indulgences that you love. (Ice cream? Pizza? Chocolate chip cookies?) The key is to know how many calories you can *afford* for that day and stay within that range.

Now you can be as lean and healthy as you want just by using the flexible diet method. No more guilt, no more stress, no more dieting failures. Your body can rest from the yo-yo, back-and-forth torture of strict dieting.

Your mind can rest as well. And that brings us to our next point.

## 2) Comparison of Your Mind:

### Strict / Fad Diets

People who are involved in the sales industry have a saying:

"The confused mind always says no."

To a salesperson, that means you must stay focused and keeps things simple. Compare this to the world of strict dieting. Did you ever enter a world that was so filled with vague terms, conflicting suppositions, and confusing information? The world of dieting and weight loss is rife with all of the above. You talk to one person who is on a specific diet, and they firmly believe that everything they are doing (down to the last stalk of celery) is the right way to go about things.

Talk to another person who is on yet another type of diet, and they are just as convinced and religious about their approach.

That is until they are either 1) miserable and bored with the whole mess, or 2) they hear about yet another diet that seems much better and more efficient than the one they're on at the moment.

Confusion reigns! And the confused mind always says no.

Confusion equates to a lack of confidence, and a lack of confidence relates to a lack of commitment. And since both of these individuals are miserable anyway, quitting becomes all that much more comfortable.

The mind and the emotions have a great deal to do with the process of weight loss. The most significant culprit in this area is guilt. Because most diets are a setup for failure, the chronic dieter is all too familiar with the agony of failing – time after time. If any success is involved – and it sometimes is – it's short-lived.

Instead of food simply being *food*, it has been transformed into an *enemy* that must be conquered. Dieters become exhausted just thinking about diet and weight loss and all the anxiety that is involved. Many times this can lead to the person seeing themselves as a loser and a failure. One who is "less than." Many begin to give up – not just on a diet but *self* as well. Depression is often the result.

Are these types of consequences worth it?

Have you ever heard of stair-step dieting? Perhaps you've experienced it, but had no name for it. What happens is this:

The dieter goes on a diet and successfully loses weight. Later that weight is gained back and *then some*. If this happens repeatedly, the accumulated effect is continued weight gain.

With it comes the shame and a state of emotional turmoil which can end up in bingeing cycles. The feeling is that they failed simply because they didn't try hard enough, or didn't have enough willpower, or didn't have what it takes to stick with it.

Again, it's a setup for failure.

## Flexible Dieting

None of the above is applicable when it comes to *flexible dieting*. The roller coaster cycle of moving from diet to diet is broken once and for all. Because you're eating what's right for you, eating your food preferences, eating foods you enjoy, the dieting-misery is out of the picture altogether. Guilt and shame are also removed.

Food becomes food again – that's as it's supposed to be in life. No longer are you in a battle with the very substance that's needed to sustain you and your health. This brings a fantastic amount of rest, peace, and freedom.

Eating the foods that are right for you and your goals and purposes, and moving away from the stress, guilt, and shame can add years to your life. As we are all aware, stress can be a silent killer, so why give it an extra place in your life over dieting?

Here's the uptake. Eat foods you like and enjoy. Balance your macronutrient intake. Restrict calories – but only moderately. Like magic, the psychological burden of trying to lose weight is gone. In fact, losing weight becomes comfortable and enjoyable. Sounds like something a person could live with for a sustained length of time, right?

Does that mean you'll never slip up? Well, you're human, aren't you? You go out to eat with friends, and you eat more than usual. Just go with the flow. No need to suffer through guilt and shame. Just work it (the possibility of occasional slip-ups) into your plan and don't fear it. (No more beating yourself up!)

Your calorie deficiency may have moved over into a calorie surplus. A modest binge is not the end of the world. Just get back on track and carry on.

If you're one who's been chained to the dieting cycle, does this sound like a different way of life? You're right. So next, let's look at *lifestyle*.

## 3) Comparison of Your Lifestyle:

## Strict / Fad Diets

The lifestyle of the habitual dieter who uses the strict dieting plans is neither pleasant nor appealing. It's a life filled with fretting and worrying, mixed in with bouts of failure, hopelessness, and discouragement.

The person caught in this trap is just that – trapped; hence, the cycles have continued for so long, and it's difficult to envision getting free of them.

The unsuccessful dieter is usually not a very happy person. In fact, many are just plain old miserable. What kind of life is that? It's not good for the one who's trying to lose weight, and it's probably not a whole lot of fun for those who are in proximity. (That would be friends, family, acquaintances, and co-workers.) What's more boring than to hear the weeping and moaning over the latest diet failure?

# Flexible Dieting

Compare this with the lifestyle of the one who has discovered the flexible dieting method. This person is allowed to go to a company dinner and not sit there and fret that their current diet does not approve everything on the *menu*. Not at all. This person can relax because she knows her macronutrient intake for the day and knows exactly what she can eat, or not eat and still be on track for meeting her goals.

This person is stress-free (no whining or complaining) and is quite enjoyable to be around.

The flexible dieting method *becomes a lifestyle*. It's a plan that can be maintained for months – and then for years. No set up for failure here. No falling off the wagon.

As you can see from what has been covered in this chapter, the differences between the strict (fad) diet and the flexible diet are many. In the next section, we want to filter out some of the myths about flexible dieting. Having the full, clear picture is essential.

# CHAPTER 4: THE
# FUNDAMENTALS OF CALORIES

*"Everything is energy, and that's all there is to it. Match the frequency of the reality you want, and you cannot help but get that reality. It can be no other way. This is not philosophy. This is physics."* – *Albert Einstein*

Weight loss is derived from universal laws at its core. There's one law in particular that explains how we lose weight. The body obeys the first law of thermodynamics. The first rule simply states that energy can neither be created nor destroyed and is often referred to as the energy balance equation (or energy balance law).

$$\Delta U = Q - W$$

## (Change in Internal Energy) = (Heat) - (Work)

This law gets the credit for how much weight we lose or gain.

A calorie, by definition, is a unit of heat energy.

If you eat more than your body requires every day, you're bound to gain weight. Gaining weight typically means the body is a **caloric surplus**. Unwanted fat stores are attributed to the excess intake of these, hopefully, delicious units of energy.

If you eat less than your body needs every day, you're going to lose weight. Losing weight is attributed to being in a **caloric deficit**.

Our bodies can also be at equilibrium, meaning our weight remains the same. In this case, the body is at a **caloric maintenance** level.

Does this mean that you can eat whatever you want while in a caloric deficit and still lose weight? Yes, it's possible but ill-advised. People who try this usually neglect specific macronutrient nourishment, which we'll discuss in more detail later on in this book.

The focus of this book is on losing weight, specifically from fat, while being in a caloric deficit and not in misery at the same time!

When the energy balance equation is applied to fitness, it simply translates to energy (foods) that enters the body and strength that leaves the body as either work (exercise) or heat.

$$\Delta E = E_{in} - E_{out}$$

## (Change in Body Weight) =

## (Energy Consumed) - (Energy Expended)

I'm of the opinion that weight should come off as fast as possible! I don't want to be guessing (eyeballing portions) and hoping I'm in a caloric deficit. I've tried that approach (the eating clean foods approach) to weight loss, and I can confirm it's a drag. There's no need to drag out the weight loss process. That approach to weight loss usually leads to people quitting because of a mix of frustration and disappointing progress.

I know one thing for certain: numbers don't lie.

A usual concern for people starting IIFYM is thinking about numbers or math. IIFYM only requires algebra gymnastics if you don't take advantage of IIFYM-friendly apps. Food tracking apps like "MyFitnessPal" (MFP) have been created to make tracking food consumption a breeze. MFP does all the heavy lifting (the math) for you! Here's an example:

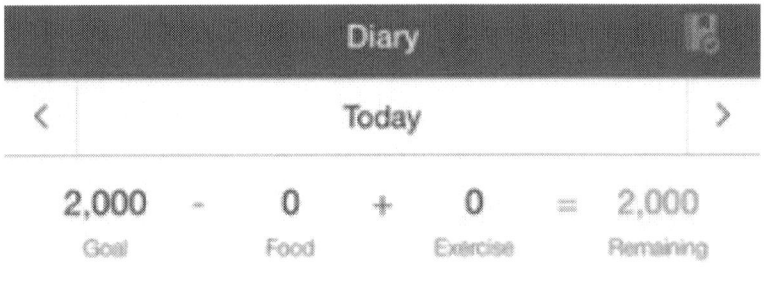

Look familiar? It's the energy balance equation in action slightly rearranged.

The easiest way to start IIFYM is by logging in what you eat with MFP. If you choose to you can track your exercise as well!

We'll be using MFP as our food tracker because it's the most highly rated and popular food tracking app available. Think of this app as the fuel gauge in your car. You wouldn't want to go on a road trip from California to Washington with your fuel gauge broken. You might make it to your destination, but you will encounter a variety of unnecessary obstacles along the way.

Knowing how much fuel is in the "tank" is imperative to losing weight promptly. MFP will be your energy fuel gauge. This handy app will give you an insight into why you're getting closer or further to your goal. Knowing your total calorie consumption carries the potential to save you time on your journey. In other words, it eliminates guessing and if you value time as I do then guessing is something you do not want to be associated with.

MFP can be used on any smart device (iPhone, Android, iPad/tablet, or on a regular computer). Most people use their smartphones to track their food intake because it's the most convenient option, namely because your phone's camera can be a barcode scanner.

I'll be showing you step-by-step examples of how to track your food, and thus your macros, on an iPhone (MFP's user interface is similar and consistent across all smart devices). Before we get started, it's time for you to take your first action step!

## Out Your Body's Daily Calorie Requirement

In addition to knowing about calories, the flexible dieter will know their macronutrient requirement in relation to their height, weight, and activity level.

## Once you know your body's daily calorie requirements, the next step is relatively clear-cut:

- Eat more calories = weight gain.

- Eat fewer calories = weight loss.

• Eat this amount of calories = weight maintenance.

## Why Each Main Macronutrient Matters

Before we leave this tutorial on how to calculate your macros, let's take a closer look at each of the three macronutrients and why they are essential:

## Carbohydrates

We need carbohydrates because:

• They are the body's primary source of fuel.

• Can be easily used by the body for energy.

• Provide glucose which is used by tissues and cells in the body for energy.

- The central nervous system, kidneys, brain and muscles (including the heart) must have carbohydrates to function properly.

- Carbs are essential for intestinal health and waste elimination.

## Protein:

We need protein for:

- Growth (especially significant for children, teens, and pregnant women).

- Tissue repair.

- Proper functioning of the immune system.

- Producing essential hormones and enzymes inside the body.

- Energy when carbohydrates are not available.

- Preserving lean muscle mass.

# Fats:

Fats are not the culprits most diet gurus make them out to be. In fact, good fats are needed for survival, and at least 20-35% of calories should come from good fat sources. Fats are necessary for:

. Allowing healthy growth and development.

. Providing the most concentrated source of energy to the body.

. Helping the body absorb essential vitamins such as A, D, E, K and carotenoids.

. Providing cushioning for internal organs.

. Maintaining cell membranes.

. Providing taste, consistency, and stability of foods.


A quick glance at these lists gives substance to the fact that we all need a wide variety of foods to maintain good health. By their very nature, restrictive diets will eliminate one or more of these health benefits.

In addition to the macronutrients, remember the body also needs a healthy amount of water each day and added micronutrients. Micronutrients are the trace vitamins and minerals that round out a healthy diet.

## Cardio:

So, to get the body of your dreams, do you need to partake in hours of mind-numbing cardio such as walking on the treadmill or stair climbing?

The answer to the above question is: probably not.

The primary purpose of the aerobic exercise is to increase the heart rate to burn more calories. If excess calories are not consumed, then cardio is not required, it is that simple – many professional bodybuilders are so precise with their caloric intake that they can obtain a competition level physique (3-4% body fat with masses of lean muscle) just through diet manipulation alone!

If you do, however, surpass your caloric target for the day, then cardio can be a convenient tool to offset these excess calories. But don't forget "you can't out train a bad diet." If you calculate your calories using this method, I will present to you further in this book that you will not be required to do any cardio.

I personally incorporate small amounts of cardio (in the form of high intensity intervals) into my routine to lose the last few pounds of fat instead of dropping my calories lower once I have recalculated my TDEE. TDEE and calculations will be discussed a bit later on in this book.

*Note: aerobic activities are fantastic for cardiovascular health, increasing performance in sports, speed, and agility, etc. However, that is outside the scope of this book.*

## Calories:

So what is a calorie?

A calorie is an energy source. Humans require calories to maintain life. We are continually trying to increase and decrease our caloric intake based on our goals, such as:

whether we want to slim down, gain lean muscle mass or perform a particular way of sports. If a calorie that is consumed is not utilized, it will be converted by the body and stored as fat.

Calories can come from several different macronutrient sources. These include:

- **Protein** – 4 calories per gram– protein serves as building blocks for lean muscle mass.

- **Carbohydrates** – 4 calories per gram – our bodies use carbohydrates as the primary energy source. Carbohydrates are broken down into 2 subcategories (both contain 4 cals/gram).

- **Simple carbohydrates** – these are the sugary processed carbohydrates that are found in foods such as lollies, chocolate, and fruit. Simple carbohydrates are absorbed quickly and cause a large insulin spike.

- **Complex carbohydrates** – These carbohydrates are the 'clean' slow digesting carbohydrates that are known for sustained energy. Complex carbs are found in brown rice, sweet potato, and oats.

- **Fat** – 9 calories per gram – Healthy fats are vital for bodily functions such as hormone levels. Fats are also broken down into several categories:

- **Saturated fat** – found in dairy and meat, can raise cholesterol.

- **Unsaturated fat** – found in vegetable oils, used to lower cholesterol.

- **Alcohol** – 7 calories per gram – empty calories (alcohol does not contain any macronutrients).

## Calculating Your Macronutrients

To begin your flexible diet, you need to know your daily caloric goal! Be sure to have a calculator or degree in mathematics on hand. To calculate this goal, the following formula is used (please note the slight variation in the formula for men and women):

Based on the extremely accurate Mifflin - St Jeor equation

- MEN: BMR = [9.99 x weight (kg)] + [6.25 x height (cm)] - [4.92 x age (years)] + 5

  WOMEN: BMR = [9.99 x weight (kg)] + [6.25 x height (cm)] - [4.92 x age (years)] -161

The above equation will give you your BMR – this is your Basal Metabolic Rate. In other words, the number of calories your body needs to function while at rest.

You then multiply the BMR by an 'activity variable' to obtain your TDEE (total daily energy expenditure). This Activity Factor is the cost of living, and it is based on more than just your workouts. It also includes work/lifestyle, sports and the thermogenic effect of food (necessarily the amount of energy burned in the process of digesting food).

Average activity variables are as follows:

- 1.2 = Sedentary - Little or no exercise + desk job

- 1.3-1.4 = Lightly Active - Little daily activity and light exercise 1-3 days a week

- 1.5-1.6 = Moderately Active - Moderately active daily life and moderate exercise 3-5 days a week

- 1.7-1.8 = Very Active - Physically demanding lifestyle and hard training or sports 6-7 days a week

1.9-2.0 = Extremely Active - Hard daily exercise or sports and physical job

Below are some examples of this calculation performed correctly:

Male

- 90kg male – 21 years old - 187cm tall – desk job, minimal exercise

- [9.99 90] + [6.25 187] – [4.92 21] – 5 Activity Level 1.2 = 2350 calories

- 70kg male – 18 years old - 170cm tall – physical job, lots of exercise

- [9.99  70] + [6.25  170] – [4.92  18] – 5  Activity level

  1.7 = 2852 calories

---

Female

- 65kg female – 28 years old – 140cm – desk job, minimal exercise

  [9.99  65] + [6.25  140] – [4.92  28] – 161  Activity level 1.2 = 1500 calories

- 55kg female – 18 years old – 150cm – moderately active

  [9.99  55] + [6.25  150] – [4.92  18] – 161  Activity level 1.5 = 1414 calories

Alternatively, you can use an online calculator based on the Mifflin – St Jeor equation, merely googling *"Mifflin st jeor equation calculator"* will result in several online calculators.

# Chapter 5: Goal-Based Calorie Consumption

Now that you have calculated your TDEE (Total Daily Energy Expenditure), you need to determine what your goal is. Do you want to maintain your current state? Do you want to strip fat? Do you want to pack on lean muscle?

The most significant mistake being made when deciding to lose weight is to go into starvation or 'crash' diet. Dropping to 1000~ calories per day will initially give you a period of weight loss at an impressive rate, however. This WILL cause metabolic damage (the process of your body rapidly decreasing its metabolism and the rate at which calories are burned due to the minimal amount of food it is receiving, mostly going into survival mode). Also, you guessed it: the only way to repair a damaged metabolism is to start to eat more slowly. Crash dieting is not sustainable - do not do it.

- For weight loss – consume 500 calories below your TDEE per day.

- For lean muscle gain – consume 500 calories above your TDEE per day.

- To maintain – consume the exact number of calories as your TDEE each day.

As your progress begins to slow down, it is time to re-calculate your TDEE via the same formula you used previously (listed above) as you will now find that your TDEE has changed! As you add lean mass, your TDEE will considerably increase. As you begin to lose weight, you will notice your TDEE has decreased (and, therefore, after a month you only be eating 200 calories under your TDEE instead of the 500 calories that you were initially consuming under).

> Note: I personally recalculate TDEE on a monthly basis; I recommend you do the same.

# Calorie Macronutrient Breakdown:

Now that we have determined your calorie goal, and established that you could eat whichever foods you choose to reach this magical caloric value, it is essential to develop an accurate ratio of protein, carbohydrates, and fats to consume.

For optimal performance in sports and resistance training (as well as to keep your appetite in check), I recommend consuming at least 30% of your daily calories from protein, with the remaining 70% coming from a breakdown of calories and fats.

You'll notice in the standard macronutrient splits listed below, the percentage of calories derived from fat does not drop below 20%. This is because hormones are constructed from cholesterol along with other fat molecules; decreasing the rate of fat consumed any lower can suppress your healthy hormone levels. Why is this an issue, you ask? Because these hormones drive the growth and development of your body, your metabolism, reproduction system, and mood. Low fat intake causes a deficiency in essential fatty acids and also highly increases your risk of cancer.

Although, as stated, you will lose fat by merely consuming under your TDEE calories and gain weight by eating above your TDEE, I would highly recommend following a high protein approach. If you neglect your protein intake, you will not build and retain lean muscle. Meals high in protein will also keep you feeling fuller for longer, unlike those rich in carbohydrates and fats.

*Note: When referring to a macronutrient breakdown, the order listed is Protein: Carbohydrates: Fat*

## Common macronutrient splits include:

*30P:50C:20F*
moderately high protein, high carbohydrate, low fat.
Often used when going through a mass building or 'bulking' phase.

*35P:40C:30F*

Moderately high protein, moderately high carbohydrates, higher fats than usual. This is a reasonably even split of macronutrients, and I would recommend this style of macronutrient split when maintaining your current body composition.

*40P:40C:20F*

High protein, high carbohydrates, and low fat.The most commonly used macronutrient split used by bodybuilders and fitness enthusiasts today, used for both fat loss and addition of lean muscle mass by merely adjusting the number of calories consumed.

*50P:30C:20F*

High protein, low carbohydrate, low fat.

This macronutrient split is often used for ongoing fat loss diets, as the high protein content keeps the individual feeling quite full and content between their meals. With this low level of carbohydrates, refeeds are necessary (this will be discussed further in the book).

*35P:60C:5F*

Moderate protein, high fat, minimal carbohydrates.

A diet comprised of these macronutrients is known as a 'ketogenic diet.' The primary purpose of this diet is to adjust the body to use fat as the primary stored energy source as opposed to carbohydrates – when the body enters this state (which takes several days), it is in a state of ketosis. I would not recommend following this style of macronutrient breakdown due to the previously mentioned hormone suppression that occurs with low-fat diets. Food choice is also insufficient to essentially meats, nuts and a small portion of vegetables, which defeats the purpose of flexible dieting.

---

Personal Note:

I follow a 40:35:25 macronutrient breakdown.

For example – I am currently consuming 2800 calories to trim the last bit of body fat; my daily macronutrient breakdown is 280 grams of protein per day, 245 grams of carbohydrates per day and 78 grams of fats per day.

---

# Required Macronutrients:

## Fiber

Fiber is an essential macronutrient that our body needs for aiding digestion. A 'clean eating' diet comprises lots of foods that contain high fiber content – however, while flexible dieting, it is equally essential that we meet our fiber needs.

Women need to aim for 22 – 28 grams of dietary fiber per day.

Men need to aim for 28 – 34 grams of dietary fiber per day.

There is a range of fiber supplements available on the market. However, these are (as the name suggests) only a supplement to your regular fiber intake. Foods high in fiber include whole grains, fruits, and vegetables (note: these are all forms of carbohydrates).

# Refeeds

What is a Refeed?

If you are embarking on a fat loss journey through the use of flexible dieting (or any style of dieting!), it is paramount to incorporate structured refeeds. Please note that this section is irrelevant if you intend to follow a calorie surplus to gain lean mass. A structured refeed is a 24-hour period in which you drastically alter your macronutrient breakdown after being in a calorie deficit (consuming fewer calories than your TDEE).

Why is a Refeed Essential?

A refeed will boost your metabolism and assist in restoring your Leptin hormone levels - Leptin is the king of all fat burning hormones. When in a calorie deficit, your metabolism will drop (meaning fewer calories are being burnt), plus your leptin hormone levels will drop in the attempt by the body to spare body fat. This is a safety mechanism put in place for the body.

We need to understand that our body is resistant to change, no matter what our current body composition is - our body does not want to change. The human body does not want to lose fat; it simply wants to survive. Consuming below your TDEE (Total Daily Energy Expenditure) will force your body to slow down your metabolism, resulting in a lower caloric intake to continually burn body fat.

As the metabolism begins to slow and Leptin levels drop, it becomes a lot harder to burn excess body fat. Therefore, including a refeed day into your diet will encourage your body to burn fat at a consistent rate.

The leaner you are, the more often you will need to refeed; lower body fat = lower leptin levels. This is based on body fat percentage; you will learn how to calculate this in the section below.

| Body fat Percentage | Frequency of Refeed |
|---|---|
| Over 20% | Monthly |
| 15 - 20% | Fortnightly |
| 10 - 15% | Weekly |
| Under 10% | Twice Weekly |

Refeed Frequency

Please refer to the following table for refeed timing:

Carbohydrate Intake During a Refeed

On your structured refeed day, I recommend you leave your protein and fat intakes the same as any other day. However, double your carbohydrate intake for this 24 hour period. This will put you slightly over your maintenance calories for the day, but it will have long-term benefits (as discussed above).

Here is an example of my regular caloric intake:

2800 calories (500 below my TDEE)

280 grams of protein

245 grams of carbohydrates

78 grams of fats

Here is my typical caloric intake on a structured refeed day:

3780 calories (580 calories above my TDEE)

280 grams of protein

490 grams of carbohydrates

78 grams of fats

As we have previously addressed, a carbohydrate is a carbohydrate – you can derive these extra carbohydrates from whichever source you choose, it does not matter whether they are simple or complex. On a refeed day, I typically indulge in oats, ice cream, pancakes, bananas and pasta as these are all very rich in carbohydrates.

# CHAPTER 6: MEAL TIMING

I'm sure you've heard this before: to achieve your fitness goals, you need to eat a more significant number of smaller meals (for example 5 – 6 meals a day). This, along with clean eating, is preached heavily by nutritionists and personal trainers.

What if I told you meal frequency and nutrient timing doesn't matter at all? Or that eating 6 times a day will not affect your metabolism or metabolic rate? That you can eat carbs right before bed and you won't gain fat?

Upon first thinking about this, it may sound like I'm making this all up. Surely consuming food before sleeping will be stored as fat as you are not actively exercising to utilize these calories. However, our body does not operate like this – it is continually looking at the bigger picture, the calories/ macronutrients we consume over a 24 or 48-hour period. Your body is frequently breaking down and repairing itself, storing and oxidizing nutrients.

It's hard to instantly change your beliefs on an aspect of fitness that is preached continuously, but a paradigm shift is required – individuals spend far too much time stressing over the timing of their meals and how many they consume a day rather than focusing on the most important aspect of dieting.

<u>Eat what you want, when you want - as long as you hit your caloric goal.</u>

A study on the "Effect of the Pattern of Food Intake on Human Energy Metabolism" states:


**Lose Fat, Not Weight**


Before we delve deeper into the following sections, it is imperative we clarify weight loss and fat loss.

Weight loss is one of the most lucrative topics in existence. The majority of people claim that they want to lose weight or fat, interchangeably switching between both of these hot keywords – little do they know there is a big difference between the two.

*Weight Loss* refers to your total body weight; this is the sum of your bones, muscles, organs, water, and fat.

*Fat Loss* refers to the amount of fat you are carrying on your body, measured as a percentage of your total body weight.

When weight loss is discussed, I'm sure you can now see that this is indeed a reference for people wanting to lose fat. In the 'tracking progress' section below, I will show you how to accurately assess your fat loss progress if this is indeed your goal.

The primary issue when discussing 'weight loss' is how unreliable it is. Your total weight fluctuates daily based upon stomach, bowel and bladder content, water loss and retention; with a large carbohydrate intake, water is bound (this is why a low/no carb diet will initially give you an impressive decrease in weight, as you no longer retain anywhere near as much water). Muscle loss and gain, as well as fat loss and gain, also play a major role. Researchers refer to those who lose weight easily but find it harder to gain weight to be 'spendthrift' with those that can gain weight easily but have more of an issue losing weight to be 'thrifty' – this ties in with the body types

## Sustainability of Flexible Dieting

How sustainable is flexible dieting? Can you continuously eat delicious foods of your choice and consistently make progress?

Of course! Flexible dieting/IIFYM will continue to work as long as you are reaching your calorie/macronutrient goal and recalculating your TDEE on a regular basis. However, if you intend to follow a flexible dieting approach for an extended period, there are a few points that must be addressed

- Continually deriving your carbohydrates from simple sugars can lead to adverse health conditions, such as increased blood sugar levels (which can lead to diabetes), high blood pressure and more. I regularly have check-ups with my local general practitioner to ensure all my levels are within a healthy, normal range.

- If you do not include a variety of vegetables within your diet, I continue to stress the importance of getting your daily vitamins and minerals via the supplementation of a multivitamin.

- Ensure you are reaching your fiber intake for the day before you consume all of your carbohydrates.

- You should time your meals based on your workout schedule. You should consume a pre-workout meal 60 – 90 minutes before training, comprised of protein and complex carbohydrates for energy. Immediately after your workout is the ideal time to consume simple carbohydrates (chocolate, lollies, etc.) to refuel your glycogen stores (which are now depleted from stressful exercise). You will not make any additional weight loss/gains by doing this. However, for overall energy and recovery pre-and post-workout nutrition are vital.

- The primary purpose of IIFYM is to achieve your desired body composition. It does not emphasize overall heart or organ health, unlike clean eating.

Therefore, from a health perspective, it is worth adapting the theory and principles behind IIFYM into your diet, as opposed to eating sugar ridden lollies as your primary source of carbohydrates.

# CHAPTER 7: MFP FEATURES FOR IIFYM SUCCESS

*"You'll never change your life until you change something you do daily. The secret of your success is found in your daily routine." – John C. Maxwell*

At the end of the day, it's the people who regulate their food intake who have the most significant successes in their fat loss journeys. I don't even consider logging in food a hassle anymore. Once you start seeing progress with IIFYM, the once upon a time "hassle," gets transmuted into a habit.

The price of doing what everyone else does is simple: little to no weight loss progress and return to old habits. Of course, it's easier just to grab some healthy food and cook it, or in some cases, heating up leftovers. This is the approach most people take.

I want you to have long-term success, and to do that, in fitness or any other area of life, it requires obtaining new habits. While reading this chapter, remember that you're learning a process that'll take you to your end goal if you commit.

## Saving Time with Meal Entries

When I first started tracking my food I didn't want to think about numbers every time I was going to eat. What I realized was that measuring foods (in ounces, grams, cups, tablespoons etc.) wasn't as bad when you created a meal plan which was tailored just for you, a topic that's coming up soon. Combine a meal plan, with MFP's logging features, and tracking becomes extremely easy.

MFP makes tracking what you eat easily because it upkeeps a history database, similar to an internet browsing history, of the foods you've eaten in the past. Having a database, built into MFP, is great because it quickly retrieves past food entries and allows it to be easily added to any meal you choose.

A great shortcut on MFP is the *Smart Copy* feature which has the potential to remove any hassle from food tracking. The *Smart Copy* feature will save you the most time if you have a meal plan, or consistently eat the same meals every day. It quickly lets you add what you ate yesterday (or X amount of days before) to the present day's corresponding meal. You do this with one quick swipe of a finger.

Take the following steps to enable the *Smart Copy* feature. The steps should also be a great example of how this process looks like.

**Step 1:** Select ••• *More*

**Step 2:** Select Turn On Smart Copy

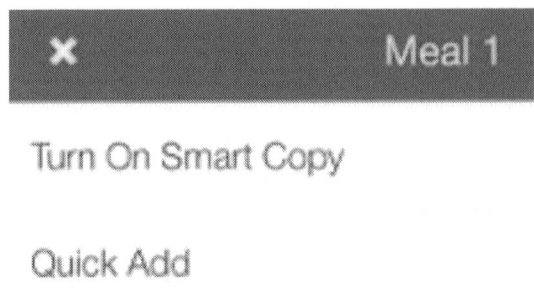

**Step 3:** Swipe right to add

It's as simple as that. You can enable, or disable, this feature for any meal you'd like. Depending on your real situation, you might need to adjust what gets copied. Sometimes you might want to add or remove a particular food that gets copied from the day before. You're able to approve what gets copied and what doesn't.

## Meal Plans: The Easiest Way to Use MFP

Meal plans require a little bit of initial work to set up. But once you've got one, it's done, and it's like putting yourself on fat burning auto-pilot mode.

Consider it a better approach than having to ask yourself "Okay consistently... what am I going to eat today?" every few hours of every day. Take the time to create a meal plan and liberate yourself from such decisions.

Take a look at a meal plan I created for myself:

# Meal 1:

- Chicken breast (~8-9 oz. uncooked weight)
- Red potatoes (~ 15-16 oz.)
- 2 whole eggs
- 85 grams of broccoli (weighed frozen)
- Light Butter (14 grams)
- Dark Chocolate (1-2 Squares)

# Meal 2:

- Chicken Breast (~8-9 oz. uncooked weight)
- Lentil Beans (1 cup)
- Brown Rice (1 cup)
- 1 egg
- 85 grams of broccoli (weighed frozen)
- Light Butter (7 grams)

# Meal 3:

- Low Fat Cottage Cheese (1/2 cup)

- Whey Protein (1 scoop)

- Peanut Butter (4 grams)

- Quaker Oats (10 grams)

- Banana (40 grams sliced)

- Stevia Packet

- Walden Farm Zero Calorie Chocolate Syrup

As you can see, I only eat three meals a day and skip breakfast. This is an intermittent fasting example of meal planning, but a meal plan nonetheless. By the way, IIFYM and Intermittent fasting complement each other handsomely, but that a topic for a future book.

The great thing about meal plans is that you can tailor them to your needs. Whether that's three, four, five, or six meals a day! Your pick of foods is up for grabs as long as you hit your daily macros. Be strategic about the foods you pick. Make sure to include nutritiously dense foods in each of your meals to ensure satiety. You can fit treats into your daily macro limit, be aware that you'll most likely not feel full if they're massively spread throughout your meal plan. I recommend having your daily treat alongside one of your meals.

An easy way to a create a meal plan is to brainstorm the foods you like to eat and distribute them amongst the number of meals you'd like to eat every day. You can use grocery items you already have at home and cross-check the nutritional values (macros). Simply scan or search foods in MFP and create a meal plan that fits your macros. Creating a meal plan takes time, so set aside some time to complete this task. I usually start this process by writing down my plan and then transferring the final meal plan into a nice spreadsheet.

## Eating Out (Nutrition Info. Available)

Just because you set a fitness goal to improve your health and lifestyle doesn't mean you have to eliminate eating out.

Such a tradeoff would be absurd. On days, I know I'm going out to eat, I like to plan.

MFP has an impressive feature called, *Create a New Food* under *My Recipes & Foods* in the main menu.

You can take advantage of using this feature by doing some quick Google research on the place you're going to be dining at. The *Create a New Food* feature allows to you input the calories (and macros) you find from your Google research. This natural process involves Googling nutrition information and configuring what you see in your MFP diary.

Unless you want to ask for nutrition information at the restaurant, then I suggest you do some quick research before going out to eat (for simplicity, I'll be using the word *restaurant* to describe traditional restaurants and fast food places alike).

Do you have a restaurant in mind?

Good, take a look at the example below. It's an example of me creating a new meal entry, in MFP, for a Chipotle Mexican Grill meal:

**Step 1:** Google: *"restaurant"* + *nutrition*

**Step 2:** Select the nutrition calculator option if available

Nutrition Calculator - Chipotle
https://www.**chipotle**.com/**nutrition**-calculator ▾ Chipotle Mexican Grill ▾
Chipotle Mexican Grill, USA, Canada and UK. Burritos, Tacos and more. Food With
Integrity

*Note: Some restaurants will only have nutrition facts and not a calculator. This varies from website to website*

**Step 3:** Choose Your Meal

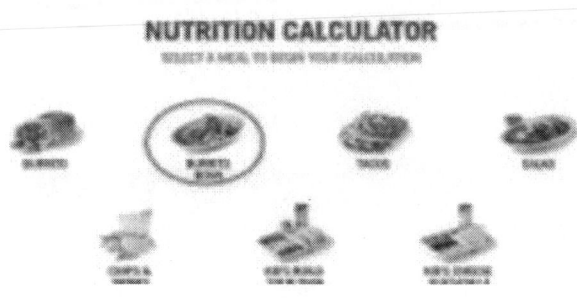

**Step 4:** Select Your Ingredients

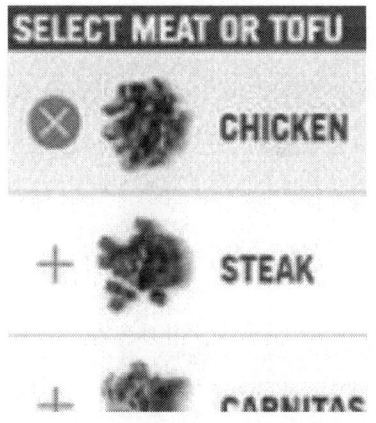

**Step 5:** Check the Nutrition Total: Calories and Macronutrients

## TOTALS

| | |
|---|---|
| SERVING SIZE (OZ) | 16.5 |
| CALORIES | 650 |
| CALORIES FROM FAT | 210 |
| TOTAL FAT (G) | 22.5 |
| SATURATED FAT (G) | 11 |
| TRANS FAT (G) | 0 |
| CHOLESTEROL (MG) | 163 |
| SODIUM (MG) | 1385 |
| CARBOHYDRATES (G) | 61 |
| DIETARY FIBER (G) | 15 |
| SUGAR (G) | 4 |
| PROTEIN (G) | 44 |

**Step 6:** Create a New Food in MFP and fill in the details

**6a)**

| More |
|---|
| 👑 Premium |
| 👤 My Profile |
| 🎯 Goals |
| 🏆 Challenges |
| 🍎 Nutrition |
| 🏆 My Recipes & Foods |

**6b)**

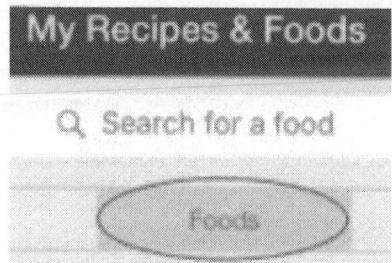

**6c)**

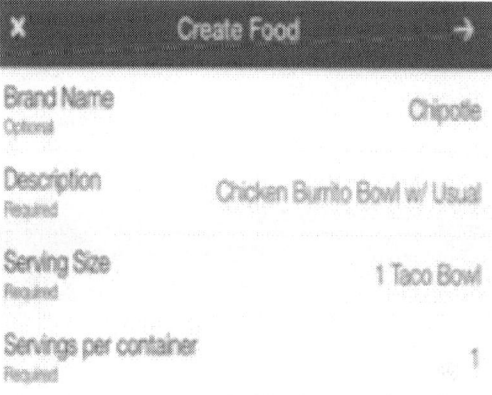

**Step 7:** Fill in Nutrition Info. (from Step 5)

**7a)**

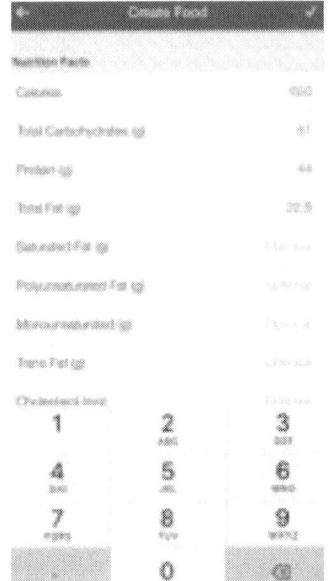

**7b)**

## Add Nutrient Information

Your diary is more accurate when you
add nutrient details.

No Thanks  |  Add Details

**7c)**

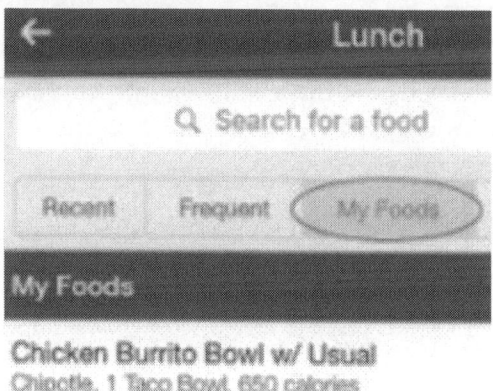

Chicken Burrito Bowl w/ Usual
Chipotle, 1 Taco Bowl, 650 calories

This is great, now I can add a chicken burrito bowl from Chipotle to any of my meals, whenever I choose to eat there again. Next time I eat out at Chipotle, I won't have to redo the process above! You can use this method for any restaurant meal you enjoy.

Unfortunately, not every restaurant provides easy-to-use online nutrition calculators like Chipotle's website. In most cases, they don't need to. You usually know what you're getting, and expecting, in most cases.

For example, In-N-Out Burger can easily be searched in MFP's database (use Method 1 from Ch. 3). I usually go with a "double-double burger." I search MFP for: *"double-double*

*in n out."*

This method of eating out looks like this:

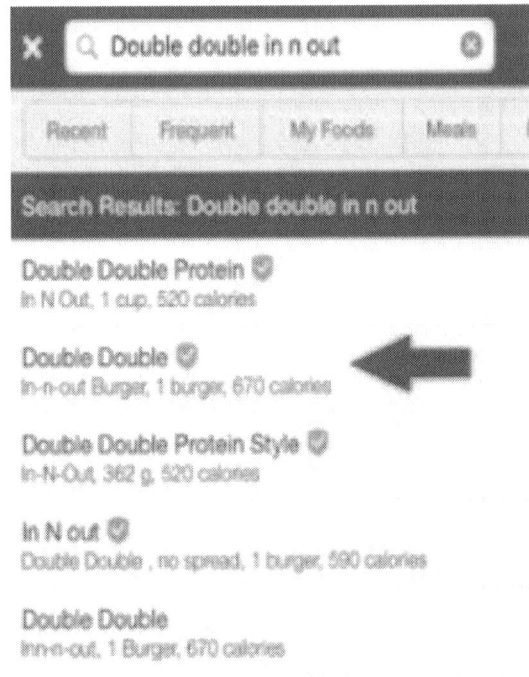

then

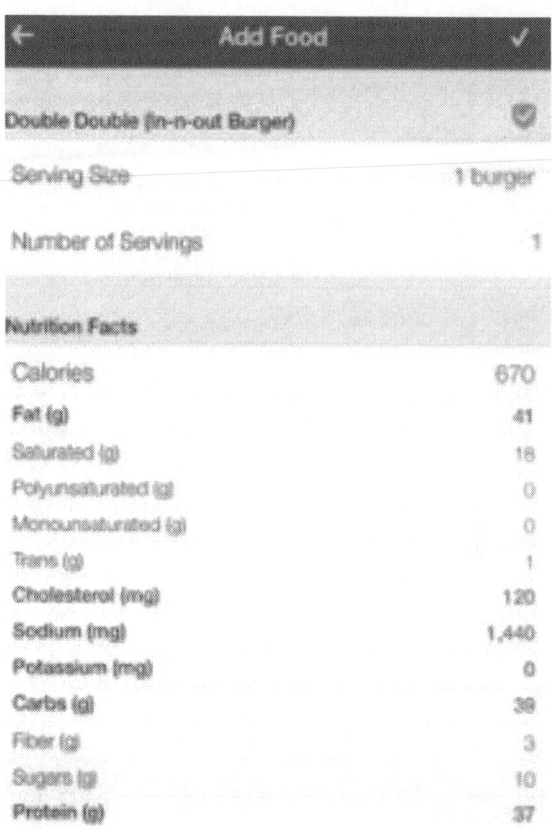

Not too bad right? If you felt like adding fries with that, you know what to do.

## Eating Out (Nutrition Info. Unavailable)

There are times when restaurants don't provide nutrition information online or offline. This can be the case if you're in one of those, delicious "hole in the wall" type spots of town. Another occasion could be that you're at a more formal restaurant, eating at a social gathering, like a barbecue, or eating a hot dog at a ball game. Is there a way to log this in? Well, yes and no, we can use a rough estimate approach.

Let's use a traditional restaurant scenario; you've ordered a lean cut of steak and mashed potatoes. You noticed that the steak is 10 ounces according to the menu. The weight of mashed potatoes wasn't given. It's time to bring out MFP and search generic entries for both foods while you wait for the food to be served.

| Lunch | 595 cal |
|---|---|
| Steak<br>Steaks, 10 ounce | 475 |
| Mashed Potatoes W/ Gravy<br>Generic, 1 cup | 120 |
| + Add Food | ••• More |

You can tailor this method to any scenario you encounter. Of course, it's not going to be 100% accurate, but "ballpark" will be good enough for these situations.

There's no reason to skip out on a restaurant meal because nutrition information wasn't available! Just do your best to stay within your caloric deficit, remember that's the key. Some flexible dieters don't log in foods, in such occasions, because it's not worth the hassle, for one, and two, because they know the food they're consuming won't push them over maintenance. Sure their caloric deficit percentage won't be ideal, but they will not gain weight.

If you go overboard, it's not the end of the world. One day of over spillage won't kill you. However, if you make eating out a consistent habit, it might add up to very little visual progress, or worse, set you back for days.

As you can see, there's no silver bullet when it comes to eating out. There are different strategies for different scenarios at best. Being prepared for, at least, one of them makes it easier to gauge your intake and lessens the chances of gaining fat by making you aware of what you're consuming.

## Moderation is Key

*"If one oversteps the bounds of moderation, the greatest pleasures cease to please." – Epictetus*

Everything in moderation. Will you never eat cookies or go out to a fast food joint again? I doubt it; well, I know I couldn't at least. This is why I treat myself to these foods in moderation.

Moderation, in my experience, is having a maintenance day once a week. A day where I eat at equilibrium where I know, I'm not going to be losing or gaining weight. The scale the next morning might rise, but I know it's temporary water weight, glycogen, and most importantly I know it's not weighted from fat.

I usually have maintenance days on Fridays or Saturdays. Eating at maintenance once a week will not hinder your weight loss efforts. I believe they're psychologically necessary. They're almost like reward days if you think about it.

Before I started IIFYM, I used to binge on fast foods. The scenario went like this:

Full>satisfied>bloated>uncomfortable>" wow why did I do that." And on some occasions, I drank alcohol on the same nights! This is a common combination that leads to fat gain.

It's worth noting that 1 gram of alcohol is equivalent to 7 calories.

When I go out to eat, I stay within my daily macro budget as going out to eat on a maintenance day is just a bonus. What another type of diet allows for this?! Rest assured, as long as it's not a daily habit, fast food is not off limits.

# CHAPTER 8: TRACKING YOUR PROGRESS

*"Success is nothing more than a few disciplines,*

*practiced every day."*

*– Jim Rohn*

Body composition describes the percentage breakdown of the amount of muscle, body fat, bone and water our bodies are composed of.

You're going to want to be proactive by tracking numbers associated with your weight and waist circumference. You want to understand your body composition as much as possible throughout your fitness journey to always know if you're headed in the right direction.

To make sure you're on the right track, losing fat, not wasting time, and doing so in a healthy manner, measuring your progress is essential. In the words of Lord Kelvin, a physicist & engineer (who determined the correct value of a Kelvin (273°C)), "If you cannot measure it, you cannot control it." Measuring is a part of progressing and should be a weekly habit, and can even be a daily habit.

There are two primary tools, outside of MFP, you're going to use to measure your progress and chances are you have these devices lying around somewhere.

## Weight and Pictures

The weight scale is the iconic progress tracker when it comes to weight loss. Although it doesn't provide us with the whole story, on our progress, it's still useful.

Keep in mind that weight fluctuates depending on the time of day you weigh yourself. Throughout your journey, you might weigh yourself one day and seem to have lost a pound, and the next you're back at square one, or sometimes even a pound heavier. This is normal and is nothing to stress over. Everyone encounters this issue when they're in a caloric deficit, and you're not alone.

Many factors have an impact on weight fluctuations. A few of these factors are water retention, bowel movements, and glycogen storage. To get the most accurate scale reading, we're going to measure by the weekly averages, not days. Weigh yourself at the same time every day. Make sure to do this first thing in the morning, on an empty stomach, as well as, after using the restroom to get the most accurate reading. At the end of every week take the average of your readings and note that it doesn't have to be every day of the week.

MFP can handle tracking your daily weight measurements.

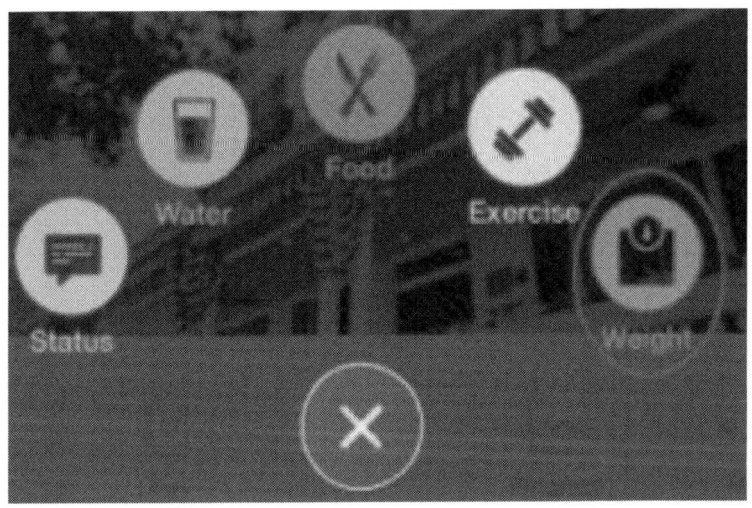

MFP also gives you the option to take photos, which I highly recommend, when you go to record your weight.

Pictures, along with mirror reflection analysis, will help you get a better understanding of how you're progressing. It's also really great to look back at your old photos and compare them with the new you! MFP lets you compare photos side by side, detailing both the date you took the picture and how much you weighed on that day.

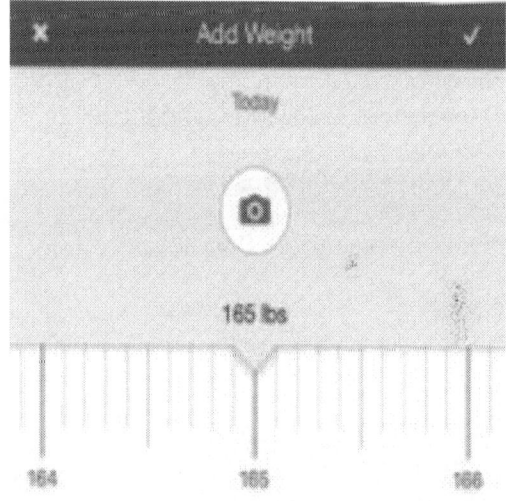

If you'd like to see your progress, at a glance, you can do so by selecting *Progress* in MFP's lower menu.

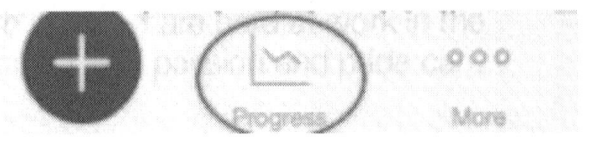

Selecting this will take you to a page where you can view the progress you've made. It allows you to see your past progress in a graph mode. The graph shows data points of your weight entries (the y-axis) and the date you recorded them (x-axis). You can also adjust the time frame of this graph by weeks, months, and years.

This is a handy feature that is much better than keeping a separate journal and having to record every day in my opinion manually. Be consistent, and your graph will end up looking like a beautiful fluctuating mess (you'll see what I mean soon).

## Waist

The second method of tracking progress is using a waist tape measure. A tape measure is arguably more revealing than the scale because you can potentially have a smaller weight on the same day the weight on the scale is stagnant. Along with photos, it can be a determining factor, to check, if you've genuinely gained weight or if your body is just retaining water. For those reasons, it's a good idea to measure your waist, just above the belly button, after you weigh in.

To get the most accurate reading, relax and don't suck in your tummy. Breathe as you usually would and get a reading.

MFP will track waist measurements in the same fashion it follows weight.

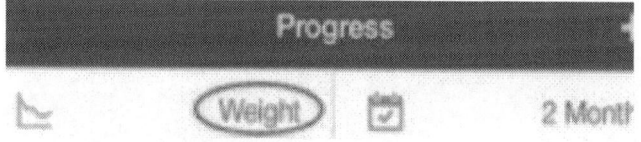

You can change the progress settings by switching "Weight" to "Waist" to record your waist measurement.

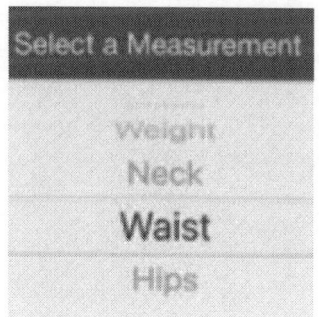

# BONUS CHAPTER - FLEXIBLE DIETING RECIPES

The next 3 pages contain a few of my favourite flexible dieting meals. These are easy to fit into your daily macronutrients and very easy to make. I am far from a master chef, so if I can make these - so can you. I eat these meals on a regular basis.

If you enjoy these recipes, be sure to stay tuned for a dedicated recipe and protein smoothie book, which I will be releasing shortly.

## Protein Power Pizza

Description:

A delicious miniature protein pizza, this recipe can be altered to suit your personal preference. However, this is a great base to work with.

Ingredients:

Wholemeal Pita Bread

Tomato Paste

Whole Chicken

Baby Spinach

Tomatoes

Mushroom

Cheese (if desired)


Method:

- Spread tomato paste over wholemeal pita bread base

- Cut up chicken and place on pizza (1 whole chicken = 6 pizzas)

- Cover pizza with spinach, mushroom, and tomato

- Place pizzas in over on 200 degrees Celsius (392F) for 20 minutes

Macronutrients

Per pizza

Protein: 50g

Carbohydrates: 45G

Fat: 5G

425 calories

# Premium Protein Cheesecake

Description:

Delicious protein cheesecake, this cheesecake can be made in different variations simply by altering the flavour of protein used (change vanilla to chocolate and add some topping) or stick with vanilla and add some berries.

Ingredients:

340 grams (12oz) fat-free cream cheese280 grams (10oz) plain Greek yogurt

2 eggs

2 tbsp. stevia

¼ cup of milk

2 scoops whey protein

1 tsp vanilla extract

Dash of salt

Method:

- Preheat oven to 160 degrees Celsius (320F)

- Soften cream cheese in a large mixing bowl

- Add eggs and stevia, proceed to mix

- Add the remaining ingredients

- Mix all ingredients for 3 minutes

- Pour mixture into baking pan lined with parchment paper

- Bake at 160 degrees Celsius (320F) for 20 minutes then adjust to 90 degrees Celsius (194F) for an hour

- Place in fridge for 5 hours to cool

- Serve with toppings if desired

*Macronutrients*

per 225 grams (8oz) slice

40g protein

15g carbohydrates

2g fat

238 calories

# Mad Monkey Protein Smoothie

Description:

A thick and delicious chocolate smoothie that packs a punch!
Great for increasing your energy level before a workout.

Ingredients:

2 scoops chocolate whey protein

100ml skim milk

1 banana

1 tbsp. peanut butter

1 tbsp. coffee

1 cup ice

Method:

- Place all ingredients in a blender or magic bullet
  and blend for ~20 seconds

- Enjoy!

Macronutrients:

55g protein

32g carbohydrates

15g fat

401 calories

# CONCLUSION

Dieting is something we all talk about. People often search for the perfect diet, following each new fad as it appears, hoping that this will be the one that will allow us to make progress. Unfortunately, there is much more chance of failure with each 'fasting' or 'caveman diet' that we try... not necessarily because they don't work, but because they are not something which we can follow over a prolonged period. Any diet that leaves you feeling deprived is almost certainly bound for failure, as is one that goes you bored with the foods that you are allowed to eat. The ONLY way to successfully make progress towards your goals is to change the way you eat.

Flexible dieting will allow you to incorporate the foods you love into your diet in moderation and still make weight loss progress (or lean muscle gains, depending on your goal). There will no longer be the need to stress about what you can eat when you go out socially as certain foods are no longer labeled as 'bad' or 'fattening.' Now that you know how to calculate and track your daily intake, you can look forward to your next meal instead of dreading the thought of having to consume tasteless boiled vegetables.

For me, flexible dieting is the key to living a balanced, healthy lifestyle in a body I am proud to own. Setting goals and achieving them with the help of flexible dieting creates new found confidence in the individual which, in turn, motivates you to stay true to the path of the ongoing journey – it is the flow of positive, constant progression. You're either spiralling up or spiralling up.

I hope you enjoyed reading this book as much as I enjoyed creating it for you. I would like to wish you the best of luck with your flexible dieting, so go out there and achieve your goals!

# Final Words

Thank you again for purchasing this book!

I really hope this book is able to help you.

The next step is for you to **join our email newsletter** to receive updates on any upcoming new book releases or promotions. You can sign-up for free and as a bonus, you will also receive our "*7 Fitness Mistakes You Don't Know You're Making*" book! This bonus book breaks down many of the most common fitness mistakes and will demystify many of the complexities and science of getting into shape. Having all this fitness knowledge and science organized into an actionable step-by-step book will help you get started in the right direction in your fitness journey! To join our free email newsletter and grab your free book, please visit the link and signup: **www.hmwpublishing.com/gift**

Finally, if you enjoyed this book, then I would like to ask you for a favor, would you be kind enough to leave a review for this book? It would be greatly appreciated!

Thank you and good luck in your journey!

# About the Co-Author

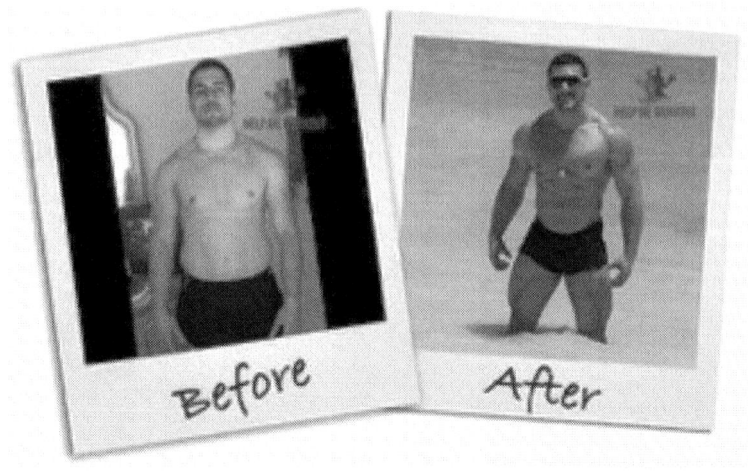

My name is George Kaplo; I'm a certified personal trainer from Montreal, Canada. I'll start off by saying I'm not the biggest guy you will ever meet and this has never really been my goal. In fact, I started working out to overcome my biggest insecurity when I was younger, which was my self-confidence. This was due to my height measuring only 5 foot 5 inches (168cm), it pushed me down to attempt anything I ever wanted to achieve in life. You may be going through some challenges right now, or you may simply want to get fit, and I can certainly relate.

For me personally, I was always kind of interested in the

health & fitness world and wanted to gain some muscle due to the numerous bullying in my teenage years about my height and my overweight body. I figured I couldn't do anything about my height, but I sure can do something about how my body looked like. This was the beginning of my transformation journey. I had no idea where to start, but I just got started. I felt worried and afraid at times that other people would make fun of me for doing the exercises the wrong way. I always wished I had a friend that was next to me who was knowledgeable enough to help me get started and "show me the ropes."

After a lot of work, studying and countless trial and errors. Some people began to notice how I was getting more fit and how I was starting to form a keen interest in the topic. This led many friends and new faces to come to me and ask me for fitness advice. At first, it seemed odd when people asked me to help them get in shape. But what kept me going is when they started to see changes in their own body and told me it's the first time that they saw real results! From there, more people kept coming to me, and it made me realize after so much reading and studying in this field that it did help me but it also allowed me to help others. I'm now a fully certified personal trainer and have trained numerous clients to date who have achieved amazing results.

Today, my brother Alex Kaplo (also a Certified Personal Trainer) and I own & operate this publishing venture, where we bring passionate and expert authors to write about health and fitness topics. We also run an online fitness website "HelpMeWorkout.com" and I would love to connect with by inviting you to visit the website on the following page and signing up to our e-mail newsletter (you will even get a free book).

Last but not least, if you are in the position I was once in and you want some guidance, don't hesitate and ask... I'll be there to help you out!

Your friend and coach,
**George Kaplo**
Certified Personal Trainer

# Download another book for Free

I want to thank you for purchasing this book and offer you another book (just as long and valuable as this book), "Health & Fitness Mistakes You Don't Know You're Making", completely free.

Visit the link below to signup and receive it:

**www.hmwpublishing.com/gift**

In this book, I will break down the most common health & fitness mistakes, you are probably committing right now, and I will reveal how you can easily get in the best shape of your life!

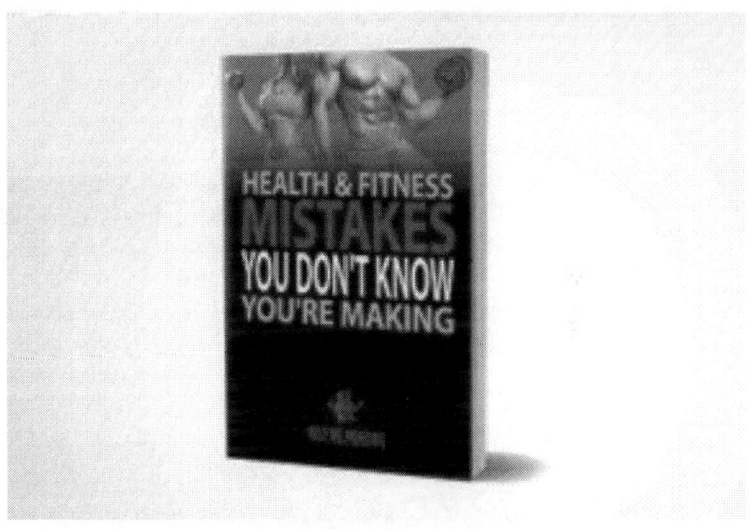

In addition to this valuable gift, you will also have an opportunity to get our new books for free, enter giveaways, and receive other valuable emails from me. Again, visit the link to sign up:

**www.hmwpublishing.com/gift**

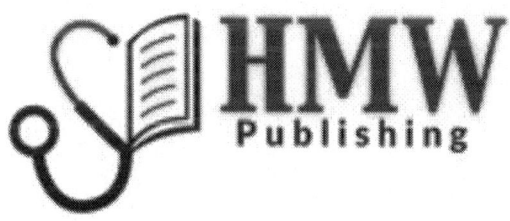

For more great books visit:

**HMWPublishing.com**

Made in the USA
Lexington, KY
17 April 2019